12 THINGS THAT INDIVIDUALS WITH POWERFUL MINDS DON'T DO:Toughen yourself up and break harmful mental habits.

Betty J. Thompson

TABLE OF CONTENT

Chapter 1

Don't give away your power

What are the ways you cede authority to others? Although you may believe otherwise, there are several ways in which we cede our control. For instance:

Never be afraid to change when you want the approval of someone else.

Anytime you say yes when you really mean no, or no when you really mean yes

When another person has the capacity to aggravate you,

When you seek someone else to provide you with all of the solutions,

If you see yourself attempting to impress others,

When you put up with unhealthy partnerships

When you keep quiet out of concern about hurting someone

When you don't think well of or accept who you are

Ignore the things that are beyond your control.

Though I'm sure you get the concept, there are a lot more options. Recognize when you are losing your power and decide to take back control of your life.

Chapter 2

Don't shy away from change

Making a change in your life seems easy. The solution to losing weight is to increase your physical activity and improve your diet. Alternatively, you might just leave your job and look for a new one if your employment isn't fulfilling you.

But it's challenging to make such adjustments. It is a totally different thing to know something and put it into practice.

Of course, there are instances where change is initially simple—those exceptions to the norm. Perhaps you have a strong desire to alter your spending patterns. However, after the first two weeks, the plan loses its excitement, which makes it difficult for you to stay motivated and follow through.

Prior to making any changes in your life, you must first recognize the areas in which you are resistant to change.   change becomes ingrained in the lives of many individuals. And in the end, it saps their mental fortitude. It seems easy enough to change your life. The solution to losing weight is to increase your physical activity and improve your diet. Alternatively, you might just leave your job and look for a new one if your employment isn't fulfilling you.

But it's challenging to make such adjustments. There are, of course, certain exceptions to the rule—those instances in which change is initially simple. However, knowledge and action are two very different things. Perhaps you have a strong desire to alter your spending patterns. However, after the first two weeks, the plan loses its excitement, which makes it difficult for you to stay motivated and follow through.

Prior to making any changes in your life, you must first recognize the areas in which you are resistant to change. Avoiding change becomes ingrained in the lives of many individuals. And in the end, it saps their mental fortitude.

The ten indicators that you resist change are as follows:

1. Any alterations to your routine cause you a great deal of concern.
2. Every time you make a change, it's difficult for you to maintain.
3. You consider the adjustments you would want to make, but you convince yourself that now is not the appropriate moment to make such changes.
4. You convince yourself that making changes is pointless since they won't stick.
5. You use statements like "I'd like to exercise more, but my spouse won't go to the gym with me" as justifications for why you are unable to make changes.

6. You persuade yourself that your terrible behaviors are OK since they aren't "that bad."

7. It simply feels too frightening to consider moving outside of your comfort zone.

8. You find it difficult to adjust when your friends, family, or employer make changes that impact you.

9. You don't act differently even when things are difficult because you don't believe that things will get better with change.

10. It's tough for you to remember the last time you set out to improve yourself.

You're not alone if any of those phrases describe you. We all have concerns about our capacity to handle the stress that comes with change.

The good news is that everybody can bring about constructive change. You can find the courage to accomplish your objectives, regardless of whether you want to kick a harmful habit or start over in a new chapter of your life.

Chapter 3

Don't focus on things you can't control

To what extent are you driven to put an end to the time-wasting contemplation of uncontrollable things?

Whether we like it or not, the brain is trained and conditioned by repetition. When your thoughts stray to uncontrollable matters, remind yourself of your hard-won successes or your desired goals.

Create several short-, medium-, and long-term strategies. Attempt to be prepared, efficient, and well-organized.

I would role-play both parts in my head before every significant encounter. For each criticism, I would have a well-thought-out argument and a rebuttal. I made extensive use of similes and metaphors.

It is so easy to start thinking incorrectly when things don't go our way. Our thoughts and places become uncontrollable as we drift. Worried about all the awful things that might occur next, we begin to dwell on everything that isn't going our way. We become imperceptible to the world around us and forget how we contribute to it. Today, this is still possible. There are good days and bad days for everyone in our group, even if we are battling a worldwide pandemic. We strive to be productive and have a pleasant attitude on our good days.

We wallow in our despair on bad days, trying to project what we think the future holds. Fear and helplessness creep in as we picture it and then begin to live it. Dr. Shannon Irvine, a neuropsychologist, says that's because "thoughts really do create your emotions." Brain connections are made after thought fires before emotion. That link will begin to run automatically if you click it enough times. When we think negatively, we experience negative emotions because thoughts ignite before emotions do. That being said, there is a workaround. I make every effort to return my focus to the most crucial element of all whenever I catch myself drifting from a positive to a pessimistic vision. Three questions are what I ask myself:

Why am I worried? What I can control How can I address the things that are most important to me? Considerations that center on our sphere of influence give us power and elicit favorable feelings. The Roman and Stoic philosopher Epictetus explained this reason in a Manual for Living. One key idea that must be understood clearly in order to achieve freedom and happiness is that not everything is in our control. To detect and distinguish between things that are external to me and outside of my control and those that are related to decisions I can make for myself is the main task in life. One fundamental idea that guides our approach to life is this one:

Should we cede our power to forces beyond our control or hold onto it and focus our efforts on the things within our control? I deliberately make an effort to swim out of anxiety when my mind tricks me and pulls me into one. Moreover, I refocus my ideas and lift them into a happier frame of mind.

Chapter 4

Don't worry about pleasing everyone

We would all have a different response if asked why we desire to satisfy others in the first place. This explains why individuals with varying enneagram numbers may have distinct motivations for their actions. An underlying dread of being rejected or an aversion to unpleasant circumstances might exist. It's possible that people-pleasing conduct is a learned one.

It is dangerous to attempt to please everyone. Remember that when you commit to saying yes to anything, you're also likely to say no to something else that you may care about more. We could even get engrossed in trying to win someone over for the wrong reasons. The never-ending hustle may easily lead to burnout, which can have an impact on our stress levels, our ability to achieve our objectives, and our personal lives. Being always polite is a waste of time;

it leaves you open to manipulation, and it's just not a sustainable way of living. Make sure you scroll up to listen to the podcast as we go into further depth.

It's not important to please everyone. You have no control over the happiness of another person. Make sure you're continually going back to discover what drives your desire to satisfy people. We discuss having courageous discussions in this episode, even with your employer! Here are some more things to consider:

Regularly examine your motives.

Engage in courageous dialogue.

Establish and maintain sensible limits.

Recall that you are not in charge of controlling other people's feelings.

Don't be disrespectful; instead, project confidence.

Chapter 5

Don't fear about taking calculated risk

All people have naturally experienced fear at some point in their lives. It's a defense system that keeps us safe and helps us stay out of harm's way. But when fear gets out of control, it may prevent us from realizing our full potential and accomplishing our objectives. It's crucial to develop your ability to face fear and take measured risks because of this.

Don't look back at the past. Taking calculated risks entails analyzing the advantages and disadvantages of a given option and selecting it after careful consideration. It's about acting with purpose and strategy rather than just taking chances or acting irresponsibly.

Avoid repeating the same mistakes by using the following advice to conquer fear and take measured risks:

1. Determine the cause of your fear. Recognizing the root of your fear is the first step towards conquering it. Is it fear of not knowing what to do, fear of failing, or dread of what other people may think? You can start addressing your fear once you know what's generating it.
2. Acknowledge failure: Taking chances always leads to failure. It's important to keep in mind that failure is a chance to develop and learn, rather than the end of the path. Consider your mistakes and what you might do better the next time. This will provide you with more understanding and confidence while taking on risks in the future.

Chapter 6

Don't give up after the first failure

You won't find it simple to accomplish your ambitions. You can't expect to wake up one day and find yourself in possession of everything you've ever desired, just because you wanted it so much. Your desires are insufficient. Your good intentions fall short. What's going to get you to success is what you do. You must exert yourself, put in the hours, shed tears and blood, and put in the effort.

When it comes to your greatest aspirations, you cannot continue to put them off. You can't keep promising yourself that you'll begin working toward your objectives tomorrow. Now is the ideal moment to get started. Make no excuses without holding back. In any case, findings won't appear right away. You should go ahead and make a head start today, as it will take you a long time to complete the tasks you have set out to perform. You'll succeed more quickly the earlier you start.

It goes without saying that you won't succeed on your first try. You're going to be unsuccessful. Rejection is going to happen to you. You will commit a gazillion tiny and major errors. You can't let your fear of failing stop you, since it's an essential step on the path to success. You cannot achieve your goals without making mistakes first. It's necessary to attempt, make errors, grow from them, and try again. Up until you eventually get the outcomes you've been looking for, you need to keep repeating that cycle.

When your desire is strong enough, you persevere beyond your first setback. You don't give up because things are too difficult. You don't think you're meant to spend the rest of your life in one location. You maintain your self-confidence.

It's common to question your abilities after failing at anything. It's common to wonder whether you've been squandering your time. It's reasonable to wonder about the various routes you may choose. However, you can't let your thoughts linger on such issues for too long. You cannot presume that you are flawed since everyone on earth has committed comparable errors. Recall that those who achieve extraordinary success in your industry didn't get there the first time either.

Failure won't deter you for very long if you want something so passionately. You'll quickly get back up and give it another go. You couldn't live with yourself if you gave up on your dreams; therefore, you won't let them pass you by. It is your duty to pursue your aspirations. However, until you make the commitment, make the necessary effort, push beyond your fear of failing, and take calculated chances, you will never be able to realize those aspirations.

Remind yourself that you will not achieve your goals without making some errors, and see every setback as a teaching opportunity. Thank God you had the chance to try and fail. Thank God you have the chance to develop.

Chapter 7

Don't dwell on the past

The past, whatever it was, is no more. It is imperative that you focus on the present moment since there is nothing you can do to alter the past. It is difficult to resist the temptation to get caught up in the past. However, you need to focus on what is going on for you right now if you want to succeed in life. Whether it was good or bad in the past, you might be drawn to thinking back on it. In any case, you have to let it go because there is only one way to live: in the present. If you are looking back on the past out of regret, you must understand that there is no turning back on what you have already done. Reliving the past comes with a lot of drawbacks. Among them is ill health. It's likely that your memories of the past are not joyful and optimistic. Your health may be steadily destroyed by negative ideas. According to studies, people who often reflect on the past are less healthy than those who live in the present.

Chronic stress, anxiety, sadness, sleeplessness, obesity, and anorexia may all be caused by living in the past. You are always exhausted, which makes it difficult for you to focus at work and take advantage of all the little joys life has to offer. It's time to let go of all that has occurred in the past if you recognize it.

Chapter 8

Don't make same mistake over and over again

It's likely that you aren't entirely aware of the reasons behind your errors or that you're not doing enough to prevent them from occurring in the future. Another reason you might be making these mistakes is that you might be dealing with underlying psychological or personal problems, like low self-esteem, impulse control, or a lack of self-awareness. One way to start addressing this problem is to start journaling about the mistakes you make, the circumstances around them, and your feelings and thoughts at the time. You may use this to find trends and triggers that could be causing you to make the same errors over and over again. Seeking the advice of a therapist or counselor may also be beneficial. They can assist you in creating plans for dealing with underlying psychological or personal problems and enhancing your capacity for learning from your errors.

First and foremost, you must have faith—not in yourself, but in the fact that you are a human being, and humans have the ability to do the seemingly impossible.

You have power over everything.

Your thoughts, feelings, and emotions... Until you have confidence in yourself, everything will undoubtedly remain under your control.

When you develop a strong sense of self-love and faith, you will undoubtedly learn from your errors.

How can one develop self-belief?

Positive outlooks are the source of faith.

You mentioned, buddy, that you make mistakes frequently and can't recognize them until it's too late.

That way, at least you can recognize your errors rather than committing them mindlessly like others do.

You were therefore in a position to recognize your weakness. That is truly amazing. Half of your work is done. That's a constructive mindset.

What is causing you to make the same errors repeatedly?

It is important to remember that "everyone has a baseline behavior" that changes or evolves over time.

By using the term "baseline behavior," I intend to convey that...

We frequently pick up new skills, read a variety of ideas and proverbs, observe various types of people, events, and situations, and are then inspired or motivated to modify our behavior in response to that specific inspiration.

To illustrate, let us say that we try to recognize the opportunities and chances we have to develop and decide to work a little harder than we do every day if we see a young person our age performing manual labor as part of his daily routine or working as a salesperson in any retail market. However, that resolve fades after a few days or weeks until a fresh one appears. That is, we revert to our initial behavior.

In a similar vein, you acknowledge your errors but continue to make them since they will eventually return to your normal behavior.

It is rather typical for anybody to act in this way.

Furthermore, you are not at all meant to lose confidence.

It requires perseverance, self-assurance, tenacity, passion, and a slogan.

How can you change your ingrained behavior?

It isn't exactly simple to have a shift in your basic behavior.

- It demands patience.
- You need to fully adjust your everyday routine since this daily pattern is the source of your baseline behavior.
- You should treat your mind with notions everyday that look inspirational to you so that your mind will be used to such surroundings.

Mistakes are the nature of humans. No innovation, no creativity, is done without errors.

Whatever the error may be related to interpersonal connections, studies, or personal conduct, you may remove them.

Don't resent other people's success.

Mentally strong individuals can recognize and applaud other people's accomplishments in life. They don't become envious or feel deceived when others outperform them. Instead, they know that achievement comes with hard work, and they are eager to work hard for their own opportunity at success.

Envy is probably one of the deadliest hazards to any form of relationship. Miserable, insecure individuals are naturally envious, which stops them from interacting with others. Learn to enjoy others' successes. Even if it's not your personal triumph, you have a reason to feel happy.

Chapter 9

Don't believe the world owes you anything.

You have no assurances for your health, safety, food, housing, happiness, love, or anything else. You were born into this world to fend for yourself. For these reasons, people established families, communities, and societies in order to support one another and thereby increase our own chances of surviving and living. Take advantage of every opportunity and assist those in your immediate vicinity in order to survive and live. Remember that you must forge your own path in life and that others won't help you simply because you believe you deserve it. It implies that no one has to do anything for you and that you have to earn your keep. It really only implies that you should express more gratitude for what you already have.

The adage "the world doesn't owe you anything" kind of implies that you have to give something in order to be entitled to get anything in return. Allow me to illustrate with two examples:

Unless you have shown more work ethic, superior qualifications, and merit than other candidates for the same position, your manager does not owe you a promotion. Until you behave in a manner that makes you worthy of their respect, your neighbors do not owe you any. You don't owe anyone confidence or trust; you have to earn it. This saying is about things that are similar to these.

Chapter 10

Don't expect immediate result

We all like instant gratification as humans. Our brains are wired that way. We prefer to be informed as soon as possible about the effectiveness of our actions and whether we should make any changes. As we know, there are downsides to living a life of impatience and expecting immediate results:

Not having enough patience

Overestimate one's own capabilities

Trim the edges.

unrealistic anticipations

negative conversation

Not ready for what lies ahead

Make sure to tune in as we go into further detail about this in the episode! When we overestimate our abilities and then become frustrated that we weren't able to complete the task, this is one of the facts that can surprise us. We discuss strategies and pointers to consider during the planning stage. These tactics will happen on the front end and help tremendously on the back end. So tune into the podcast episode!

Chapter 11

How to practice patience

Don't expect immediate results. So, now what? We recognize that we can't always have our expectations satisfied quickly. Here are a few solid things we talk about in the podcast and how you can simply weave this into what you're currently doing in your day-to-day life:

Practice postponing gratification.

Remember your why?

Celebrate the tiny victories.

Create a strategy to reject temptation.

Deal with emotions in a healthy way.

Pace yourself properly.

Practice self-control and self-discipline.

All of these small tips will take you miles down the road. This will help set you up for success as well as boost your self-esteem. If you're getting annoyed with feeling impatient, call in your wise advice. They can assist, take you through, troubleshoot, and support you along the way.

Chapter 12

Maintaining mental strength

Our mental power is challenged all the time. You may lose your job or be struggling with the death of a loved one.

But what precisely is "mental strength"?

"When we talk about mental strength, what we're actually talking about is emotional resilience, which is the ability to cope with stress and challenges in a healthy way.

And mental strength, or resilience, is distinct from mental health.

"When some people hear the terms mental strength or resiliency, they may think it means the absence of mental illness, but that is not the case," explains Duke. "Many people with mental illness have learned to manage their condition in a healthy way. They have developed emotional resilience and are in good mental health. In a similar vein, an individual can be emotionally resilient and have poor mental health without having a history of mental illness.

Duke offers techniques for strengthening your mental toughness and overcoming hardship.

What is the definition of mental toughness?

The ability of a person to effectively handle difficulties, pressures, and stressors is known as mental strength or emotional resilience.

Increasing your mental toughness can help you live a more fulfilling life and guard against mental health problems in the future.

Why does that matter?

When you strive toward your goals, your mental toughness can help you feel less afraid of failing. It can also be beneficial during difficult times or after a loss. It's how you handle particular circumstances and how fast and efficiently you bounce back.

Over time, you can strengthen your mental defenses. The secret is to exercise self-care, create healthy coping mechanisms, and cultivate an understanding inner dialogue.

Going through difficult experiences helps us develop our emotional resilience as well, according to Duke. It's important to reflect and give yourself credit for overcoming adversity. I advise my customers to identify their strengths and areas for future improvement.

Techniques for enhancing mental toughness

Do you want to focus on increasing your resilience? Duke provides these tactics.

Recognize your emotions.

Throughout the day, be sure to pause and assess your own performance, advises Duke. Do you have anxiety? Upset? Happy?

"Just to be able to check in with yourself and name your feelings is so important," adds Duke. "Because without that mental check-in, you can't start to give yourself more of what you might need."

Practice being self-compassionate.

If you're scared you insulted an in-law or weren't as patient with your kid as you intended to be, consider practicing self-compassion.

The idea is to silence your inner critic and be nice and compassionate with yourself the way you would a friend.

"Practice talking to yourself, not in a critical way, but in the way that you would talk to someone who you really care about and when they are facing a problem," says Duke. "And extend yourself that same love and compassion."

Assess your challenge.

Faced with a challenge? Take a deep breath and ask yourself whether this is a serious tragedy or an inconvenience.

"We often interpret inconveniences as catastrophes," argues Duke. "Making that distinction can be helpful. Because if it's an inconvenience, then you can start to problem-solve and brainstorm. Consider all the numerous instances in your life when you were able to effectively resolve issues.

Make incremental progress toward your desired avoidance.

You tend to put off doing things you don't want to do when you're unhappy or worried. You could also put things off. (Hello, overview of the job.)

However, Duke advises working on making baby steps toward the activity or scenario rather than avoiding it completely. Could you set aside an hour every day to make that presentation?

According to Duke, "taking small steps will help to alleviate anxiety as well as improve your mood and self-esteem."

Practice being aware.

Recalling and engaging in mindfulness exercises is a wonderful idea when you're feeling tense or nervous. Allow yourself time to relax and consider your responses.

To remain present, try box breathing or a one-minute meditation.

According to Duke, "learn strategies that help you be more present." "It can be very beneficial to learn to breathe and to be present through your breath."

Externalize your emotions.

Don't suppress your emotions if anything is upsetting you. Focus on communicating assertively to put those sentiments into words.

Duke says, "The practice of naming your feelings and communicating them effectively, as well as having a supportive and empowering social circle, is really important. You can do this through journaling, therapy, or talking to your best friend."

Continue living a healthy lifestyle.

Exercise, a balanced diet, and getting enough sleep are all factors that contribute to a healthy lifestyle and may support emotional resilience.

"I don't think you can be emotionally or mentally strong without following a regular sleep schedule. You should also cut back on how much news and social media you consume."

The relationship between mental toughness and general health

Your mental toughness or resilience may impact performance, relationships, productivity, motivation, and decision-making.

According to Duke, "we know that having good mental health can help reduce the risk of dementia, heart disease, and cancer."

She continues, "But don't worry if you need to review your mental strength toolkit."

Duke says, "It's never too late to learn effective strategies." You may make a commitment to studying constructive coping mechanisms and putting them into practice. Developing these skills is something you may do in therapy, with a friend, or on your own at any time.

www.ingramcontent.com/pod-product-compliance
Lightning Source LLC
Chambersburg PA
CBHW071011260726
48661CB00007B/2905